THE COMPLETE TYPE 2 DIABETIC COOKBOOK FOR BEGINNERS

Essential guide to 2000-days of delicious low-carb and sugar-free diabetic friendly recipes for type diabetes and newly diagnosed, with a 31-day meal plan

Marcus Baron

Table of Contents

COPYRIGHT © 2023

CHAPTER ONE

Understanding Type 2 Diabetes and Nutrition

Introduction to Type 2 Diabetes: Causes, Symptoms, and Management

Type 2 diabetes is a chronic metabolic disorder characterized by high blood sugar levels resulting from insulin resistance and relative insulin deficiency. It accounts for the majority of diabetes cases worldwide and is often associated with lifestyle factors such as poor diet, sedentary behavior, and obesity.

Causes

The exact cause of type 2 diabetes is multifactorial and involves a complex interplay of genetic, environmental, and lifestyle factors. Genetics play a significant role, with individuals having a family history of diabetes being at higher risk. Additionally, factors such as obesity, physical inactivity, poor diet (high in refined sugars and saturated fats), and advancing age contribute to the development of insulin resistance and eventual diabetes.

Symptoms

Symptoms of type 2 diabetes can vary but commonly include increased thirst, frequent urination, fatigue, blurred vision, slow wound healing, and recurrent infections. Many individuals with type 2 diabetes may not experience noticeable symptoms initially, leading to delayed diagnosis and increased risk of complications.

Management

Management of type 2 diabetes aims to control blood sugar levels, prevent complications, and improve overall quality of life. This typically involves a combination of lifestyle modifications, medication, and regular monitoring.

Lifestyle modifications include adopting a healthy diet, engaging in regular physical activity, maintaining a healthy weight, and avoiding tobacco use. Medications may be prescribed to lower blood sugar levels, improve insulin sensitivity, or reduce the risk of complications. In some cases, insulin therapy may be necessary to adequately control blood sugar levels.

The Role of Nutrition in Type 2 Diabetes Management

Nutrition plays a fundamental role in the management of type 2 diabetes, as dietary choices directly impact blood sugar levels, insulin sensitivity, and overall health. A well-balanced diet can help stabilize blood sugar levels, reduce the risk of complications, and improve overall well-being.

Basics of Healthy Eating for Type 2 Diabetes

Adopting a healthy eating plan is essential for managing type 2 diabetes effectively. The following principles form the foundation of a healthy diet for individuals with diabetes:

1. Carbohydrate Management

Carbohydrates have the most significant impact on blood sugar levels and should be managed carefully. It's essential to focus on consuming complex carbohydrates that are high in fiber, such as whole grains, legumes, fruits, and vegetables, as they have a slower effect on blood sugar levels compared to refined carbohydrates. Monitoring portion sizes and spacing carbohydrate intake throughout the day can help stabilize blood sugar levels.

2. Glycemic Index

The glycemic index (GI) is a scale that ranks carbohydrate-containing foods based on their effect on blood sugar levels. Foods with a low GI release glucose slowly into the bloodstream, resulting in more stable blood sugar levels. Choosing foods with a low or moderate GI can help manage blood sugar levels more effectively. Examples of low-GI foods include whole grains, legumes, non-starchy vegetables, and most fruits.

3. Protein Intake

Protein plays a crucial role in managing blood sugar levels and promoting satiety. Including lean sources of protein such as poultry, fish, tofu, legumes, and nuts in meals and snacks can help stabilize blood sugar levels and prevent overeating. It's essential to balance protein intake with carbohydrates and fats to maintain overall macronutrient balance.

4. Healthy Fats

Including healthy fats in the diet can help improve insulin sensitivity and reduce the risk of heart disease, which is common in individuals with type 2 diabetes. Sources of healthy fats include avocados, nuts, seeds, olive oil, and fatty fish. Limiting saturated and trans fats found in fried foods, processed snacks, and high-fat dairy products is important for overall heart health.

5. Fiber-Rich Foods

Fiber is beneficial for individuals with type 2 diabetes as it helps regulate blood sugar levels, promote satiety, and improve digestive health. Including plenty of fiber-rich foods such as fruits, vegetables, whole grains, legumes, and nuts in the diet can help control blood sugar levels and reduce the risk of complications such as cardiovascular disease and obesity.

6. Meal Timing and Portion Control

Spacing meals evenly throughout the day and practicing portion control can help prevent large fluctuations in blood sugar levels and promote better glycemic control. Eating smaller, more frequent meals and snacks can also help regulate appetite and prevent overeating. It's essential to pay attention to portion sizes and avoid oversized servings, especially of high-calorie foods.

7. Hydration

Staying hydrated is important for overall health and can help regulate blood sugar levels. Drinking an adequate amount of water throughout the day can help prevent dehydration, promote satiety, and support optimal metabolic function. Limiting sugary beverages such as soda, fruit juice, and sweetened tea or coffee is important for controlling blood sugar levels and reducing calorie intake.

Conclusion

Managing type 2 diabetes requires a comprehensive approach that includes regular physical activity, medication management, and dietary modifications. Nutrition plays a central role in diabetes management, and adopting a healthy eating plan can help stabilize blood sugar levels, reduce the risk of complications, and improve overall quality of life. By focusing on carbohydrate management, choosing nutrient-dense foods, and practicing portion control, individuals with type 2 diabetes can achieve better glycemic control and enjoy better health outcomes.

CHAPTER TWO

Essential Kitchen Tools and Ingredients

Stocking Your Kitchen with Diabetes-Friendly Staples

Maintaining a well-stocked kitchen with diabetes-friendly staples is essential for preparing nutritious meals and managing blood sugar levels effectively. Here are some must-have items to keep in your pantry, refrigerator, and freezer:

1. Whole Grains: Stock up on whole grains such as brown rice, quinoa, oats, and whole wheat pasta. These are rich in fiber, which helps regulate blood sugar levels and promote satiety.

2. Legumes: Beans, lentils, and chickpeas are excellent sources of protein, fiber, and complex carbohydrates. They can be used in soups, salads, stews, and side dishes to add texture and flavor to meals.

3. Fresh Produce: Fill your refrigerator with a variety of fresh fruits and vegetables. Opt for colorful options like leafy greens, berries, citrus fruits, carrots, and bell peppers, which are packed with vitamins, minerals, and antioxidants.

4. Lean Protein Sources: Choose lean protein sources such as skinless poultry, fish, tofu, tempeh, and low-fat dairy products.

Protein helps stabilize blood sugar levels and promotes muscle health.

5. Healthy Fats: Stock up on sources of healthy fats such as olive oil, avocados, nuts, and seeds. These fats are beneficial for heart health and can help improve insulin sensitivity.

6. Herbs and Spices: Enhance the flavor of your dishes with herbs and spices instead of relying on salt or sugar. Fresh herbs like basil, cilantro, and parsley, as well as spices such as cinnamon, turmeric, and ginger, can add depth and complexity to your meals without extra calories or sodium.

7. Low-Sodium Broth or Stock: Keep low-sodium vegetable, chicken, or beef broth on hand for soups, stews, and sauces. It adds flavor to dishes without excess salt.

8. Sugar-Free Condiments: Choose sugar-free or low-sugar condiments such as mustard, hot sauce, salsa, and vinegar for added flavor without the extra carbohydrates.

9. Whole Grain Flour and Baking Ingredients: Use whole grain flour, almond flour, or coconut flour for baking instead of refined white flour. Stock up on baking essentials like baking powder, baking soda, vanilla extract, and unsweetened cocoa powder.

10. Sugar Substitutes: If you enjoy sweetening your foods or beverages, opt for natural sugar substitutes like stevia, erythritol, or monk fruit sweetener. These alternatives provide sweetness without causing spikes in blood sugar levels.

Must-Have Kitchen Equipment for Easy Cooking

Having the right kitchen equipment can make meal preparation easier and more efficient, especially when managing a condition like diabetes. Here are some essential tools every diabetes-friendly kitchen should have:

1. Measuring Cups and Spoons: Accurately measuring ingredients is crucial for portion control and managing carbohydrate intake. Invest in a set of measuring cups and spoons to ensure you're using the right amount of ingredients in your recipes.

2. Food Scale: A digital food scale is helpful for measuring ingredients by weight, especially for items like fruits, vegetables, and meats. It allows for precise portioning and helps you track your carbohydrate intake more effectively.

3. Non-Stick Cookware: Non-stick pots, pans, and skillets require less oil or cooking spray, making them ideal for preparing healthy meals with minimal added fat. They also make cleanup easier, which can save time in the kitchen.

4. Blender or Food Processor: A blender or food processor is essential for making smoothies, sauces, dips, and soups. It's also useful for chopping vegetables, nuts, and seeds quickly and efficiently.

5. Slow Cooker or Instant Pot: These countertop appliances are perfect for busy individuals who want to prepare nutritious meals with minimal effort. They allow you to set and forget recipes, making them ideal for batch cooking and meal planning.

6. Oven Thermometer: An oven thermometer ensures that your oven is heating accurately, which is essential for baking and roasting. It helps prevent overcooking or undercooking your food, resulting in better-tasting dishes.

7. Salad Spinner: Washing and drying leafy greens and fresh herbs is a breeze with a salad spinner. It removes excess moisture, ensuring that your salads are crisp and vibrant.

8. Cutting Boards and Sharp Knives: Invest in high-quality cutting boards and sharp knives for safe and efficient food preparation. Having the right tools makes chopping, slicing, and dicing ingredients easier and more enjoyable.

Understanding Carbohydrates, Sugars, and Sweeteners

Carbohydrates are one of the three main macronutrients found in food, along with protein and fat. They provide the body with energy and are found in a wide variety of foods, including grains, fruits, vegetables, legumes, dairy products, and sweets. Carbohydrates are broken down into glucose (sugar) during digestion, which is then used by the body for fuel.

Types of Carbohydrates:

Carbohydrates can be classified into three main types based on their chemical structure:

1. Simple Carbohydrates: Simple carbohydrates are composed of one or two sugar molecules and are quickly digested and absorbed into the bloodstream, leading to rapid spikes in blood sugar levels. Examples include table sugar (sucrose), honey, maple syrup, fruit juice, and refined grains like white bread and white rice.

2. Complex Carbohydrates: Complex carbohydrates are composed of multiple sugar molecules linked together in long chains. They take longer to digest and are absorbed more slowly, resulting in a gradual and steady increase in blood sugar levels. Examples include whole grains, legumes, vegetables, and fruits.

3. Fiber: Fiber is a type of complex carbohydrate that the body cannot digest. It passes through the digestive tract intact, providing bulk and promoting regular bowel movements. Fiber also helps regulate blood sugar levels by slowing down the absorption of glucose and improving insulin sensitivity. Sources of fiber include whole grains, fruits, vegetables, legumes, nuts, and seeds.

Impact of Carbohydrates on Blood Sugar:

For individuals with diabetes, monitoring carbohydrate intake is crucial for managing blood sugar levels. Carbohydrates have the most significant impact on blood glucose levels compared to protein and fat. Consuming too many carbohydrates at once or choosing high-glycemic index foods can cause blood sugar levels to spike, while spreading carbohydrate intake throughout the day and opting for low-glycemic index foods can help maintain more stable blood sugar levels.

Sugars and Sweeteners:

Sugars are simple carbohydrates that add sweetness to foods and beverages. While natural sugars found in fruits and dairy products can be part of a healthy diet, added sugars found in processed foods and sugary beverages should be limited, as they can contribute to weight gain, insulin resistance, and poor blood sugar control.

Common Types of Sugars:

- **Sucrose:** Table sugar derived from sugarcane or sugar beets.

- **Fructose:** Naturally occurring sugar found in fruits, honey, and some vegetables.

- **Glucose:** The primary form of sugar used by the body for energy.

- **Lactose:** Sugar found in milk and dairy products.

Sugar Substitutes:

For individuals with diabetes or those looking to reduce their sugar intake, sugar substitutes can be used to provide sweetness without the added carbohydrates and calories. Some common sugar substitutes include:

- **Stevia:** A natural sweetener extracted from the leaves of the Stevia rebaudiana plant.

- **Erythritol:** A sugar alcohol that provides sweetness with fewer calories and a minimal impact on blood sugar levels.

- **Monk Fruit Sweetener:** Derived from the monk fruit, this sweetener is calorie-free and does not raise blood sugar levels.

- **Artificial Sweeteners:** These synthetic sweeteners, such as aspartame, saccharin, and sucralose, provide sweetness without calories but may have a distinct aftertaste for some individuals.

Conclusion:

Understanding carbohydrates, sugars, and sweeteners is essential for managing diabetes and maintaining overall health. By choosing complex carbohydrates, monitoring portion sizes, and selecting low-sugar or sugar-free alternatives, individuals with diabetes can effectively control blood sugar levels and reduce the risk of complications. Additionally, having the right kitchen tools and ingredients on hand makes meal preparation easier and more enjoyable, enabling individuals to follow a diabetes-friendly diet with confidence and success.

CHAPTER THREE

Breakfasts to Start Your Day Right

Quick and Nutritious Breakfast Ideas for Busy Mornings

Breakfast is often considered the most important meal of the day, as it provides the body with essential nutrients and energy to kickstart the morning. However, busy mornings can make it challenging to prepare a balanced breakfast. Here are some quick and nutritious breakfast ideas that are perfect for busy mornings:

1. Overnight Oats: Prepare a batch of overnight oats the night before by combining rolled oats with milk (or a dairy-free alternative), Greek yogurt, chia seeds, and your favorite toppings such as berries, nuts, and a drizzle of honey or maple syrup. Let the mixture soak in the refrigerator overnight, and enjoy a ready-to-eat breakfast in the morning.

2. Greek Yogurt Parfait: Layer Greek yogurt with fresh fruit, granola, and a drizzle of honey or agave syrup in a jar or bowl to create a delicious and nutritious parfait. You can customize the parfait with your favorite fruits and toppings for variety.

3. Whole Grain Toast with Nut Butter: Toast a slice of whole grain bread and top it with almond butter, peanut butter, or your favorite nut butter. Add sliced bananas, berries, or a sprinkle of cinnamon for extra flavor and nutrition. This simple breakfast provides a good balance of carbohydrates, protein, and healthy fats to keep you satisfied until lunchtime.

4. Smoothie: Blend together a combination of leafy greens (such as spinach or kale), frozen fruits (such as berries or mango), Greek yogurt or protein powder, and a liquid base (such as milk, almond milk, or coconut water) to create a nutritious smoothie. You can also add ingredients like chia seeds, flaxseeds, or nut butter for added protein and fiber.

5. Egg Muffins: Prepare a batch of egg muffins filled with vegetables, cheese, and cooked lean protein such as turkey bacon or chicken sausage. Simply whisk together eggs, vegetables, and seasonings, pour the mixture into muffin tins, and bake until set. These portable egg muffins can be made ahead of time and reheated for a quick and convenient breakfast option.

6. Whole Grain Cereal with Milk: Choose a high-fiber, low-sugar whole grain cereal and pair it with low-fat milk or a dairy-free alternative. Add sliced fruit or a handful of nuts for extra flavor and nutrition. Look for cereals that contain at least 3 grams of fiber per serving and less than 6 grams of added sugar per serving.

7. Cottage Cheese with Fruit: Top a serving of cottage cheese with fresh or canned fruit (such as pineapple, peaches, or mandarin oranges) for a quick and satisfying breakfast option. Cottage cheese is rich in protein, while fruit adds natural sweetness and vitamins.

High-Fiber Breakfasts to Support Blood Sugar Control

Consuming a high-fiber breakfast is particularly beneficial for individuals with diabetes, as fiber helps regulate blood sugar levels and promotes feelings of fullness. Here are some high-fiber breakfast ideas to support blood sugar control:

1. Bran Muffins: Enjoy a bran muffin made with whole grain flour, bran cereal, and added fruits or nuts for extra fiber. Pair it with a serving of Greek yogurt or a glass of milk for added protein.

2. Veggie Omelette: Fill an omelette with sautéed vegetables such as spinach, bell peppers, onions, and mushrooms for a fiber-rich breakfast option. Serve it with a side of whole grain toast or a small serving of fruit for additional carbohydrates.

3. Chia Seed Pudding: Mix chia seeds with milk (or a dairy-free alternative) and sweetener of choice, then let it sit in the refrigerator overnight to thicken into a pudding-like consistency. Top the chia seed pudding with fresh fruit, nuts, or coconut flakes for added texture and flavor.

4. Whole Grain Pancakes or Waffles: Make pancakes or waffles using whole grain flour and add-ins like mashed bananas, grated zucchini, or blueberries for extra fiber. Serve them with a dollop of Greek yogurt or a drizzle of pure maple syrup for sweetness.

5. Quinoa Breakfast Bowl: Cook quinoa in milk (or water) and top it with sliced fruit, nuts, seeds, and a sprinkle of cinnamon for a hearty and nutritious breakfast bowl. Quinoa is a complete protein and a good source of fiber, making it an excellent choice for blood sugar control.

Breakfast Recipes That Balance Protein, Carbs, and Healthy Fats

A well-balanced breakfast that includes protein, carbohydrates, and healthy fats is important for providing sustained energy and keeping blood sugar levels stable throughout the morning. Here are some breakfast recipes that achieve this balance:

1. Avocado Toast with Eggs: Top whole grain toast with mashed avocado, a poached or scrambled egg, and a sprinkle of salt, pepper, and red pepper flakes for added flavor. Avocado provides healthy fats, while eggs offer protein, making this a satisfying and nutritious breakfast option.

2. Breakfast Burrito: Fill a whole grain tortilla with scrambled eggs, black beans, diced vegetables (such as bell peppers, onions, and tomatoes), and a sprinkle of shredded cheese. Roll up the burrito and serve it with salsa and sliced avocado for a well-rounded meal.

3. Smoked Salmon and Cream Cheese Bagel: Spread whole grain bagels with low-fat cream cheese and top them with smoked salmon, sliced cucumbers, and red onion for a delicious and protein-packed breakfast. Garnish with capers and fresh dill for extra flavor.

4. Quinoa Breakfast Bowl with Greek Yogurt: Combine cooked quinoa with Greek yogurt, sliced fruit (such as berries or bananas), nuts, seeds, and a drizzle of honey or maple syrup for a protein-rich breakfast bowl. Quinoa and Greek yogurt provide protein, while fruit adds natural sweetness and fiber.

5. Breakfast Tacos: Fill corn or whole grain tortillas with scrambled eggs, black beans, diced avocado, salsa, and a sprinkle of cheese for a flavorful and satisfying breakfast option. Serve the tacos with a side of fresh fruit or a small salad for added nutrients.

Conclusion

Starting your day with a nutritious breakfast sets the tone for a healthy lifestyle and can help regulate blood sugar levels, support energy levels, and promote overall well-being. Whether you have a few minutes to spare or need a quick grab-and-go option, there are plenty of breakfast ideas to suit your needs and preferences. By incorporating a balance of protein, carbohydrates, and healthy fats into your morning meals, you can fuel your body and mind for a productive day ahead.

CHAPTER FOUR

Balanced Lunches for Sustained Energy

Simple Salad and Wrap Recipes for Balanced Lunches

Salads and wraps are versatile and convenient options for balanced lunches that provide sustained energy throughout the day. Here are some simple recipes to try:

1. Quinoa Salad with Chickpeas and Vegetables:

- Cook quinoa according to package instructions and let it cool.

- In a large bowl, combine cooked quinoa with canned chickpeas (rinsed and drained), diced vegetables (such as cucumbers, tomatoes, bell peppers, and red onions), and fresh herbs (such as parsley or cilantro).

- Dress the salad with a vinaigrette made from olive oil, lemon juice, garlic, salt, and pepper.

- Serve the quinoa salad chilled as a refreshing and nutritious lunch option.

2. Greek Salad Wrap:

- Fill a whole grain or spinach tortilla with chopped romaine lettuce, diced cucumbers, cherry tomatoes, kalamata olives, crumbled feta cheese, and a drizzle of Greek yogurt tzatziki sauce.

- Add grilled chicken, tofu, or falafel for extra protein if desired.

- Roll up the wrap tightly and cut it in half for a portable and satisfying lunch.

3. Turkey and Avocado Wrap:

- Spread mashed avocado onto a whole grain or whole wheat tortilla.

- Layer sliced turkey breast, mixed greens, shredded carrots, sliced cucumbers, and roasted red peppers on top of the avocado.

- Roll up the wrap and secure it with toothpicks or wrap it in parchment paper for a nutritious and filling lunch on the go.

4. Asian-Inspired Quinoa Salad:

- Cook quinoa according to package instructions and let it cool.

- In a large bowl, combine cooked quinoa with shredded cabbage, shredded carrots, edamame, sliced bell peppers, and chopped green onions.

- Toss the salad with a sesame ginger dressing made from soy sauce, rice vinegar, sesame oil, honey, garlic, and ginger.

- Top the salad with toasted sesame seeds and sliced almonds for added crunch and flavor.

Protein-Packed Lunches to Keep You Full and Focused

Including ample protein in your lunch is key to staying full and focused throughout the afternoon. Here are some protein-packed lunch ideas to try:

1. Grilled Chicken and Quinoa Bowl:

- Grill or bake chicken breasts seasoned with herbs and spices such as garlic powder, paprika, and thyme.

- Serve the grilled chicken with cooked quinoa, steamed vegetables (such as broccoli, cauliflower, and carrots), and a drizzle of balsamic glaze or tahini sauce.

- Garnish the bowl with fresh herbs like parsley or basil for added flavor.

2. Lentil and Vegetable Soup:

- Cook lentils in vegetable broth with diced vegetables (such as carrots, celery, onions, and tomatoes) until tender.

- Season the soup with herbs and spices like cumin, coriander, turmeric, and bay leaves for added flavor.

- Serve the lentil and vegetable soup with a side of whole grain bread or crackers for a satisfying and nutritious lunch option.

3. Tofu Stir-Fry with Brown Rice:

- Stir-fry cubed tofu with mixed vegetables (such as bell peppers, snap peas, broccoli, and mushrooms) in a wok or skillet with a drizzle of sesame oil and soy sauce.

- Serve the tofu stir-fry over cooked brown rice or quinoa for a protein-rich and fiber-packed lunch.

4. Salmon Salad Sandwich:

- Mix canned or cooked salmon with Greek yogurt, lemon juice, Dijon mustard, chopped celery, and fresh dill or parsley.

- Spread the salmon salad onto whole grain bread or a whole wheat sandwich thin.

- Add lettuce, tomato slices, and avocado slices for extra nutrients and flavor.

- Serve the salmon salad sandwich with a side of raw vegetables or a small green salad for a complete and satisfying lunch.

Creative Lunch Ideas for Work or School

Keeping lunchtime exciting and enjoyable can help you stay motivated to eat healthily. Here are some creative lunch ideas to spice up your midday meals:

1. DIY Salad Bar:

- Set up a salad bar with a variety of toppings such as mixed greens, chopped vegetables, beans, nuts, seeds, grilled chicken or tofu, hard-boiled eggs, cheese, and dressing options.

- Allow everyone to build their own custom salads based on their preferences and dietary needs.

- This interactive lunch option is perfect for group settings and encourages creativity and variety.

2. Bento Box Lunch:

- Pack a bento box with a selection of bite-sized items such as sliced vegetables, fruit, cheese cubes, whole grain crackers, nuts, olives, and lean protein options like turkey slices or hard-boiled eggs.

- Arrange the items neatly in the compartments of the bento box for an attractive and well-balanced meal.

3. Mason Jar Salads:

- Layer ingredients for salads in mason jars, starting with dressing at the bottom, followed by hearty vegetables, grains, protein, and leafy greens on top.

- Seal the jars tightly and store them in the refrigerator until ready to eat.

- When it's time for lunch, simply shake the jar to distribute the dressing evenly and enjoy a fresh and flavorful salad.

4. Sushi Rolls:

- Make homemade sushi rolls using nori sheets, sushi rice, and fillings such as avocado, cucumber, smoked salmon, tofu, and cooked shrimp.

- Roll up the sushi tightly using a bamboo sushi mat and slice it into bite-sized pieces.

- Serve the sushi rolls with soy sauce, pickled ginger, and wasabi for a fun and delicious lunch option.

Conclusion

Balanced lunches are essential for providing sustained energy and supporting overall health and well-being. Whether you prefer salads, wraps, protein-packed meals, or creative lunch ideas, there are plenty of options to choose from to keep you fueled and satisfied throughout the day. By incorporating a variety of nutrient-rich ingredients and flavors into your lunchtime meals, you can enjoy delicious and nutritious lunches that support your health and productivity.

CHAPTER FIVE

Wholesome Dinners for Every Taste

Easy One-Pot Dinners for Minimal Cleanup and Maximum Flavor

One-pot dinners are perfect for busy evenings when you want a delicious meal without spending hours in the kitchen or dealing with a pile of dishes afterward. Here are some easy and flavorful one-pot dinner ideas to try:

1. One-Pot Chicken and Rice:

- In a large skillet or Dutch oven, sauté diced onions, garlic, and bell peppers in olive oil until softened.

- Add boneless, skinless chicken thighs or breasts to the skillet and brown on both sides.

- Stir in uncooked rice, chicken broth, diced tomatoes, and your favorite seasonings (such as paprika, cumin, and oregano).

- Cover and simmer until the rice is cooked through and the chicken is tender. Garnish with chopped parsley or cilantro before serving.

2. One-Pot Pasta Primavera:

- In a large pot, combine pasta with chopped vegetables such as bell peppers, zucchini, cherry tomatoes, and broccoli florets.

- Add vegetable broth, garlic, Italian seasoning, and a splash of white wine (optional) to the pot.

- Bring the mixture to a boil, then reduce heat and simmer until the pasta is cooked and the vegetables are tender.

- Stir in grated Parmesan cheese and fresh basil before serving.

3. One-Pot Chili:

- In a large Dutch oven or slow cooker, brown ground beef or turkey with diced onions and garlic.

- Add canned beans (such as kidney beans, black beans, and pinto beans), diced tomatoes, tomato sauce, and chili powder to the pot.

- Simmer the chili until heated through and flavors are well combined. Serve with your favorite toppings such as shredded cheese, sour cream, and sliced green onions.

4. One-Pot Lemon Garlic Shrimp and Orzo:

- In a skillet, sauté shrimp with minced garlic, lemon zest, and a splash of white wine until the shrimp are pink and cooked through.

- Remove the shrimp from the skillet and set aside.

- In the same skillet, add uncooked orzo pasta, chicken broth, lemon juice, and chopped spinach.

- Cook until the orzo is tender and has absorbed the liquid, then stir in the cooked shrimp and season with salt and pepper to taste.

Flavorful Vegetarian and Plant-Based Dinner Options

Vegetarian and plant-based dinners are not only nutritious but also packed with flavor and variety. Here are some flavorful dinner options to satisfy vegetarians and meat-eaters alike:

1. Chickpea and Vegetable Curry:

- Sauté diced onions, garlic, and ginger in a large pot until fragrant.

- Add diced vegetables such as bell peppers, carrots, potatoes, and cauliflower to the pot, along with canned chickpeas.

- Stir in coconut milk, tomato sauce, curry powder, turmeric, and garam masala.

- Simmer the curry until the vegetables are tender and the flavors are well combined. Serve over cooked rice or quinoa.

2. Stuffed Bell Peppers:

- Cut the tops off bell peppers and remove the seeds and membranes. Place the peppers in a baking dish.

- In a skillet, sauté diced onions, garlic, and mushrooms until softened. Add cooked quinoa, canned black beans, diced tomatoes, and your favorite seasonings.

- Stuff the mixture into the bell peppers and bake in the oven until the peppers are tender and the filling is heated through. Top with grated cheese if desired.

3. Lentil Shepherd's Pie:

- Cook lentils in vegetable broth until tender. Drain any excess liquid and set aside.

- In a skillet, sauté diced onions, carrots, and celery until softened. Add cooked lentils, frozen peas, and your favorite herbs and spices.

- Transfer the mixture to a baking dish and top with mashed sweet potatoes or mashed cauliflower.

- Bake in the oven until heated through and golden brown on top. Serve hot.

4. Eggplant Parmesan:

- Slice eggplant into rounds and coat them in breadcrumbs seasoned with Italian herbs and grated Parmesan cheese.

- Bake the eggplant slices until golden brown and crispy.

- Layer the baked eggplant slices with marinara sauce and shredded mozzarella cheese in a baking dish.

- Bake until the cheese is melted and bubbly. Garnish with fresh basil before serving.

Comforting Slow Cooker and Instant Pot Recipes

Slow cooker and Instant Pot recipes are perfect for busy days when you want a comforting meal waiting for you at home. Here are some cozy and delicious recipes to try:

1. Slow Cooker Beef Stew:

- In a slow cooker, combine cubed beef stew meat with diced potatoes, carrots, celery, onions, and garlic.

- Add beef broth, tomato paste, Worcestershire sauce, and your favorite herbs and spices (such as thyme, rosemary, and bay leaves).

- Cook on low for 6-8 hours or until the beef is tender and the vegetables are cooked through. Serve hot with crusty bread.

2. Instant Pot Chicken Noodle Soup:

- In an Instant Pot, combine diced chicken breasts or thighs with chopped carrots, celery, onions, garlic, and dried pasta.

- Add chicken broth, bay leaves, thyme, and salt and pepper to taste.

- Cook on high pressure for 5 minutes, then quick release the pressure. Stir in fresh parsley before serving.

3. Slow Cooker Vegetarian Chili:

- In a slow cooker, combine canned beans (such as kidney beans, black beans, and pinto beans) with diced tomatoes, chopped bell peppers, onions, garlic, and your favorite chili seasonings.

- Cook on low for 6-8 hours or on high for 3-4 hours, until the flavors are well combined and the vegetables are tender. Serve hot with toppings such as grated cheese, sour cream, and sliced green onions.

4. Instant Pot Lentil Soup:

- In an Instant Pot, combine dried lentils with diced carrots, celery, onions, garlic, canned tomatoes, vegetable broth, and your favorite herbs and spices.

- Cook on high pressure for 15 minutes, then natural release the pressure for 10 minutes before quick releasing the remaining pressure. Stir in fresh lemon juice and chopped parsley before serving.

Conclusion

Wholesome dinners come in many forms, from easy one-pot meals to flavorful vegetarian options and comforting slow cooker recipes. By incorporating a variety of ingredients, flavors, and cooking methods into your dinner routine, you can enjoy delicious and nutritious meals that satisfy your taste buds and nourish your body. Whether you're cooking for one, feeding a family, or hosting guests, there's a wholesome dinner option to suit every taste and occasion.

CHAPTER SIX

Smart Snacking Strategies

Nutrient-Dense Snacks to Tame Hunger Between Meals

Choosing nutrient-dense snacks is essential for maintaining energy levels and supporting overall health. Here are some options to help you stay satisfied between meals:

1. Greek Yogurt with Berries: Greek yogurt is high in protein and calcium, making it a satisfying snack choice. Top it with fresh berries for added fiber, vitamins, and antioxidants.

2. Hummus and Veggie Sticks: Hummus is rich in protein and healthy fats, while raw vegetables like carrots, cucumbers, and bell peppers provide crunch and fiber. Dip the veggies in hummus for a nutritious and filling snack.

3. Hard-Boiled Eggs: Hard-boiled eggs are a convenient and portable snack that's packed with protein and essential nutrients like vitamin D and choline. Enjoy them on their own or sprinkle with a pinch of salt and pepper for extra flavor.

4. Mixed Nuts: A handful of mixed nuts (such as almonds, walnuts, and pistachios) provides protein, healthy fats, and fiber to keep you feeling full and satisfied. Opt for unsalted or lightly salted varieties to keep sodium intake in check.

5. Cottage Cheese with Pineapple: Cottage cheese is a low-fat source of protein and calcium, while pineapple adds natural sweetness and vitamin C. Enjoy them together for a refreshing and nutritious snack.

6. Whole Grain Crackers with Cheese: Pair whole grain crackers with sliced cheese for a satisfying snack that provides a balance of carbohydrates, protein, and fat. Choose whole grain crackers with minimal added sugars and select cheeses that are lower in saturated fat.

Homemade Snacks That Are Low in Sugar and High in Flavor

Making homemade snacks allows you to control the ingredients and avoid added sugars commonly found in processed snacks. Here are some homemade snack ideas that are low in sugar and bursting with flavor:

1. Roasted Chickpeas: Toss cooked chickpeas with olive oil and your favorite seasonings (such as cumin, paprika, garlic powder, and chili powder). Roast them in the oven until crispy for a crunchy and flavorful snack.

2. Veggie Chips: Thinly slice vegetables like sweet potatoes, beets, or zucchini and toss them with olive oil and sea salt. Bake them in the oven until crispy for a nutritious and satisfying alternative to traditional potato chips.

3. Energy Bites: Combine rolled oats, nut butter, honey or maple syrup, and mix-ins like chia seeds, flaxseeds, and dried fruit. Roll the mixture into bite-sized balls and refrigerate until firm for a convenient and energy-boosting snack.

4. Homemade Granola Bars: Mix together rolled oats, nuts, seeds, dried fruit, and a binder like honey or nut butter. Press the mixture into a baking dish and bake until golden brown. Cut into bars once cooled for a wholesome and customizable snack option.

5. Fruit Salsa with Cinnamon Chips: Dice fresh fruit like strawberries, kiwi, mango, and pineapple and toss with a squeeze of lime juice and a sprinkle of cinnamon. Serve with homemade cinnamon tortilla chips made from whole grain tortillas brushed with olive oil and baked until crisp.

Portable Snacks for On-the-Go Convenience

When you're on the go, having portable snacks on hand is essential for staying fueled and satisfied. Here are some convenient options for snacking on the move:

1. Trail Mix: Mix together nuts, seeds, dried fruit, and dark chocolate chips for a portable and energizing snack that provides a mix of protein, healthy fats, and carbohydrates. Portion out individual servings in resealable bags for easy grab-and-go convenience.

2. Apple Slices with Nut Butter: Slice an apple and pack it with individual packets of nut butter for a portable snack that's both sweet and satisfying. The combination of fiber-rich fruit and protein-packed nut butter will keep you full and fueled for longer.

3. String Cheese: Individual string cheese or cheese sticks are convenient snacks that provide protein and calcium on the go. Pair them with whole grain crackers or a piece of fruit for added fiber and nutrients.

4. Rice Cakes with Avocado: Spread mashed avocado onto whole grain rice cakes for a portable snack that's rich in healthy fats and fiber. Sprinkle with a pinch of sea salt and red pepper flakes for extra flavor.

5. Veggie Snack Packs: Pack pre-cut vegetables like baby carrots, celery sticks, and snap peas in individual containers with hummus or Greek yogurt dip for a nutritious and convenient snack option. The combination of crunchy veggies and creamy dip is sure to satisfy your hunger between meals.

Conclusion

Smart snacking is all about choosing nutrient-dense options that provide sustained energy and support overall health. Whether you're craving something sweet, savory, or crunchy, there are plenty of wholesome snack options to suit your taste preferences and lifestyle. By incorporating a mix of homemade snacks, portable options, and nutrient-packed choices into your snacking routine, you can stay fueled and satisfied throughout the day without compromising on flavor or nutrition.

CHAPTER SEVEN

Indulgent Desserts Made Healthier

Lower-Sugar Dessert Recipes for Satisfying Your Sweet Tooth

Lower-sugar dessert recipes allow you to enjoy your favorite treats without the guilt of excessive sugar intake. Here are some recipes that satisfy your sweet tooth while keeping sugar content in check:

1. Flourless Chocolate Avocado Brownies:

- Preheat your oven to 350°F (175°C) and line a baking dish with parchment paper.

- In a food processor, combine ripe avocados, cocoa powder, honey or maple syrup, vanilla extract, eggs, and a pinch of salt. Blend until smooth.

- Transfer the mixture to the prepared baking dish and spread it evenly.

- Bake for 25-30 minutes or until set. Let cool before slicing into squares and serving.

2. Chia Seed Pudding:

- In a bowl, whisk together chia seeds, unsweetened almond milk or coconut milk, and a natural sweetener like honey or agave syrup. Add a splash of vanilla extract for flavor.

- Let the mixture sit in the refrigerator for at least 4 hours or overnight, stirring occasionally, until thickened.

- Serve the chia seed pudding with fresh fruit, nuts, or a drizzle of nut butter for added texture and flavor.

3. Greek Yogurt Cheesecake Bars:

- Preheat your oven to 350°F (175°C) and line a baking dish with parchment paper.

- In a bowl, mix together Greek yogurt, cream cheese, honey or maple syrup, eggs, vanilla extract, and a squeeze of lemon juice until smooth and creamy.

- Pour the mixture into the prepared baking dish and smooth the top with a spatula.

- Bake for 25-30 minutes or until the edges are set and the center is slightly jiggly.

- Let cool completely before refrigerating for at least 4 hours or overnight. Slice into bars and serve chilled.

4. Banana Oatmeal Cookies:

- Preheat your oven to 350°F (175°C) and line a baking sheet with parchment paper.

- In a bowl, mash ripe bananas with rolled oats, cinnamon, a pinch of salt, and optional mix-ins like dark chocolate chips or chopped nuts.

- Scoop the dough onto the prepared baking sheet and flatten slightly with a fork.

- Bake for 12-15 minutes or until golden brown and set. Let cool before enjoying.

Fruit-Based Desserts That Are Naturally Sweet and Nutritious

Fruit-based desserts offer natural sweetness along with a variety of vitamins, minerals, and antioxidants. Here are some delicious options to try:

1. Grilled Fruit Skewers:

- Preheat your grill to medium-high heat.

- Thread chunks of your favorite fruits (such as pineapple, peaches, strawberries, and bananas) onto skewers.

- Grill the skewers for 2-3 minutes on each side or until the fruit is caramelized and slightly charred.

- Serve the grilled fruit skewers with a dollop of Greek yogurt or a drizzle of honey for a simple and refreshing dessert.

2. Mixed Berry Frozen Yogurt Pops:

- In a blender, puree mixed berries (such as strawberries, blueberries, and raspberries) with Greek yogurt, honey or maple syrup, and a splash of almond milk until smooth.

- Pour the mixture into popsicle molds and insert sticks.

- Freeze the pops for at least 4 hours or until firm. Run the molds under warm water to release the popsicles before serving.

3. Baked Apples with Cinnamon and Walnuts:

- Preheat your oven to 375°F (190°C) and core apples without cutting through the bottom.

- In a bowl, mix together chopped walnuts, raisins, cinnamon, and a drizzle of honey or maple syrup.

- Stuff the mixture into the center of the apples and place them in a baking dish.

- Bake for 25-30 minutes or until the apples are tender and caramelized. Serve warm with a scoop of Greek yogurt or a sprinkle of granola.

4. Mango Coconut Chia Popsicles:

- In a blender, puree ripe mango chunks with coconut milk, chia seeds, and a squeeze of lime juice until smooth.

- Pour the mixture into popsicle molds and insert sticks.

- Freeze the pops for at least 4 hours or until firm. Enjoy these tropical treats straight from the freezer.

Guilt-Free Treats with Smart Ingredient Swaps

Guilt-free treats are made with smart ingredient swaps to reduce calories, fat, and sugar while still delivering on flavor. Here are some ideas to indulge without the guilt:

1. Avocado Chocolate Mousse:

- In a food processor, blend ripe avocados with cocoa powder, a natural sweetener like honey or maple syrup, vanilla extract, and a pinch of salt until creamy and smooth.

- Divide the mousse into serving dishes and chill in the refrigerator for at least 30 minutes before serving. Top with shaved dark chocolate or fresh berries if desired.

2. Zucchini Bread:

- Grate zucchini and squeeze out excess moisture using a clean kitchen towel.

- Mix the grated zucchini with whole wheat flour, cinnamon, nutmeg, a natural sweetener like honey or applesauce, eggs, and a splash of olive oil.

- Bake the batter in a loaf pan at 350°F (175°C) for 50-60 minutes or until a toothpick inserted into the center comes out clean. Let cool before slicing and serving.

3. Black Bean Brownies:

- Rinse and drain canned black beans and puree them in a food processor until smooth.

- Mix the pureed black beans with cocoa powder, eggs, a natural sweetener like honey or maple syrup, vanilla extract, and a pinch of salt.

- Fold in dark chocolate chips and pour the batter into a baking dish lined with parchment paper.

- Bake at 350°F (175°C) for 25-30 minutes or until set. Let cool before cutting into squares and enjoying.

4. Frozen Banana "Nice" Cream:

- Peel ripe bananas and cut them into chunks. Freeze the banana chunks until solid.

- Blend the frozen banana chunks in a food processor until smooth and creamy, scraping down the sides as needed.

- Add flavorings like cocoa powder, peanut butter, or vanilla extract if desired.

- Serve the "nice" cream immediately for a creamy and satisfying dessert.

Conclusion

Indulgent desserts can be enjoyed in a healthier way by making smart ingredient choices and incorporating nutrient-rich options like fruits, nuts, and whole grains. Whether you're craving something chocolaty, fruity, or creamy, there are plenty of guilt-free options to satisfy your sweet tooth without compromising on taste or nutrition. By experimenting with lower-sugar recipes, fruit-based desserts, and smart ingredient swaps, you can enjoy delicious treats that leave you feeling satisfied and nourished.

CHAPTER EIGHT

Flavorful Side Dishes to Complement Any Meal

Simple and Delicious Vegetable Side Dishes

Vegetable side dishes not only add color and vibrancy to your meal but also provide essential nutrients and fiber. Here are some simple and delicious vegetable side dish ideas to complement any meal:

1. Roasted Vegetables:

- Toss chopped vegetables such as carrots, bell peppers, zucchini, and broccoli with olive oil, garlic, and your favorite herbs and spices (such as rosemary, thyme, and paprika).

- Spread the vegetables in a single layer on a baking sheet and roast in the oven at 400°F (200°C) for 20-25 minutes or until tender and caramelized.

2. Steamed Asparagus with Lemon Butter:

- Steam asparagus spears until tender-crisp, then toss them with melted butter, lemon zest, and a squeeze of fresh lemon juice.

- Season with salt and pepper to taste and garnish with chopped parsley before serving.

3. Garlic Parmesan Green Beans:

- Sauté fresh green beans with minced garlic in olive oil until crisp-tender.

- Sprinkle the green beans with grated Parmesan cheese, lemon zest, and chopped fresh parsley before serving.

4. Honey Glazed Carrots:

- Steam or boil baby carrots until just tender, then toss them with a mixture of honey, melted butter, and a pinch of cinnamon.

- Cook the carrots until the glaze thickens and coats them evenly. Garnish with chopped fresh herbs if desired.

5. Caprese Salad:

- Arrange sliced tomatoes, fresh mozzarella cheese, and basil leaves on a serving platter.

- Drizzle the salad with balsamic glaze and extra virgin olive oil, then season with salt and pepper to taste.

Whole Grain and Legume-Based Sides for Balanced Nutrition

Whole grains and legumes are nutritious additions to any meal, providing fiber, protein, and essential vitamins and minerals. Here are some flavorful side dishes that feature whole grains and legumes:

1. Quinoa Pilaf with Mixed Vegetables:

- Cook quinoa according to package instructions, then toss it with sautéed mixed vegetables (such as bell peppers, onions, and peas) and chopped fresh herbs.

- Season the pilaf with a squeeze of lemon juice, salt, and pepper before serving.

2. Lentil Salad with Feta and Cherry Tomatoes:

- Cook lentils until tender, then toss them with crumbled feta cheese, halved cherry tomatoes, diced cucumbers, and a simple vinaigrette made from olive oil, red wine vinegar, Dijon mustard, and minced garlic.

- Season the salad with salt, pepper, and chopped fresh parsley before serving.

3. Brown Rice with Black Beans and Corn:

- Cook brown rice according to package instructions, then stir in canned black beans, thawed frozen corn kernels, diced red bell pepper, chopped cilantro, and a squeeze of lime juice.

- Season the rice mixture with cumin, chili powder, garlic powder, salt, and pepper for a flavorful and satisfying side dish.

4. Farro Salad with Roasted Vegetables:

- Toss cooked farro with roasted vegetables (such as butternut squash, Brussels sprouts, and red onions) and toasted nuts (such as walnuts or almonds).

- Drizzle the salad with a simple vinaigrette made from olive oil, balsamic vinegar, Dijon mustard, and honey, then season with salt and pepper to taste.

Creative Ways to Add Flavor to Your Side Dishes

Adding creative flavor elements to your side dishes can elevate any meal and make it more enjoyable. Here are some ideas to help you add flavor to your side dishes:

1. Herb Compound Butter:

- Mix softened butter with chopped fresh herbs (such as parsley, chives, and thyme) and a squeeze of lemon juice.

- Use the herb compound butter to melt over steamed vegetables, roasted potatoes, or grilled corn on the cob for an extra burst of flavor.

2. Spiced Yogurt Sauce:

- Mix plain Greek yogurt with minced garlic, lemon zest, chopped fresh mint, and a pinch of ground cumin and coriander.

- Serve the spiced yogurt sauce alongside roasted vegetables, grilled meats, or whole grain pilafs for a creamy and flavorful accompaniment.

3. Citrus Zest and Herb Gremolata:

- Combine finely grated citrus zest (such as lemon, lime, or orange) with chopped fresh herbs (such as parsley, cilantro, or basil) and minced garlic.

- Sprinkle the gremolata over cooked vegetables, grains, or fish for a bright and aromatic burst of flavor.

4. Toasted Seeds and Nuts:

- Toast a mixture of seeds and nuts (such as sesame seeds, pumpkin seeds, and sliced almonds) in a dry skillet until golden brown and fragrant.

- Sprinkle the toasted seeds and nuts over salads, grain bowls, or roasted vegetables for added crunch and nuttiness.

Conclusion

Flavorful side dishes can enhance any meal by adding variety, texture, and depth of flavor. Whether you're serving simple vegetable sides, whole grain and legume-based dishes, or creative flavor-boosting elements, there are endless possibilities to explore. By incorporating fresh herbs, spices, citrus zest, and other creative ingredients into your side dishes, you can elevate the overall dining experience and make every meal a delicious and satisfying affair.

CHAPTER NINE

Dining Out and Socializing with Diabetes

Strategies for Making Healthy Choices When Dining Out

Dining out can present challenges for individuals with diabetes, but with some strategies in place, it's possible to make healthy choices while enjoying restaurant meals. Here are some tips:

1. Plan Ahead:

- Before going to the restaurant, check the menu online if available. Look for healthier options like grilled meats, seafood, salads, and vegetable-based dishes.

- Consider calling ahead to inquire about menu options or special accommodations for dietary restrictions.

2. Watch Portion Sizes:

- Restaurant portions are often larger than necessary. Consider sharing an entree with a dining companion or ask for a to-go box to portion out a suitable serving size before starting your meal.

3. Choose Wisely:

- Opt for grilled, baked, or steamed dishes instead of fried or breaded options.

- Select lean protein sources like grilled chicken, fish, or tofu, and load up on vegetables as side dishes or main courses.

4. Be Mindful of Carbohydrates:

- Pay attention to carbohydrate-rich foods like bread, rice, pasta, and potatoes. Consider asking for whole grain options or substituting with extra vegetables.

5. Watch Sauces and Dressings:

- Be cautious of sauces, dressings, and condiments, as they can be high in added sugars and fats. Ask for sauces on the side and use them sparingly or opt for lighter alternatives like vinaigrettes.

Tips for Navigating Social Events and Special Occasions

Social events and special occasions often revolve around food, making it important to have strategies in place to navigate these situations while managing diabetes. Here are some tips:

1. Plan Ahead:

- If possible, inquire about the menu or meal options ahead of time. Offer to bring a dish that fits your dietary needs to ensure there's something suitable for you to enjoy.

2. Be Selective:

- Scan the buffet or food spread and prioritize healthier options like salads, vegetables, lean proteins, and whole grains.

- Practice portion control and limit your intake of high-sugar and high-fat items.

3. Watch Your Alcohol Intake:

- Alcohol can affect blood sugar levels and may interact with diabetes medications. If you choose to drink, do so in moderation and opt for lower-carb options like light beer, dry wine, or spirits mixed with sugar-free mixers.

4. Stay Active:

- Incorporate physical activity into social gatherings when possible. Take a walk, dance, or engage in other forms of movement to help manage blood sugar levels and offset any indulgences.

How to Communicate Your Dietary Needs Effectively

Clear communication about your dietary needs is essential when dining out or attending social events. Here are some tips for effective communication:

1. Be Confident:

- Don't be afraid to advocate for yourself and your dietary needs. Remember that restaurants and hosts are typically accommodating and willing to make adjustments.

2. Be Specific:

- Clearly communicate your dietary restrictions or preferences to restaurant staff or hosts. Provide specific details about what you can and cannot eat to ensure your needs are met.

3. Ask Questions:

- If you're unsure about menu items or ingredients, don't hesitate to ask questions. Restaurant staff should be able to provide information about preparation methods, ingredients, and potential substitutions.

4. Offer Solutions:

- When communicating your dietary needs, offer solutions or alternatives whenever possible. For example, suggest substituting a side dish or dressing to make a meal more suitable for your needs.

5. Express Gratitude:

- Show appreciation for accommodations made by restaurant staff or hosts. A simple thank you goes a long way in fostering positive interactions and ensuring a pleasant dining experience.

Conclusion

Managing diabetes while dining out and socializing requires careful planning, mindful choices, and effective communication. By following strategies for making healthy choices, navigating social events, and communicating dietary needs, individuals with diabetes can enjoy meals out and special occasions while maintaining blood sugar control and overall well-being. With practice and confidence, dining out and socializing can be enjoyable experiences that support a healthy lifestyle with diabetes.

CHAPTER TEN

Meal Planning and Preparation for Success

Practical Tips for Meal Planning and Grocery Shopping

Meal planning and grocery shopping are essential components of a successful and healthy eating routine. Here are some practical tips to help streamline the process:

1. Set Aside Time for Planning:

- Designate a specific time each week to plan your meals and create a shopping list. This could be a weekend morning or any other time that works best for you.

2. Know Your Schedule:

- Consider your schedule for the upcoming week when planning meals. Take into account busy days when you may need quick and easy options or nights when you have more time to cook.

3. Plan Balanced Meals:

- Aim to include a variety of food groups in your meals, including lean proteins, whole grains, fruits, vegetables, and healthy fats. This ensures you're getting a diverse range of nutrients.

4. Make a Shopping List:

- Use your meal plan to create a shopping list of all the ingredients you'll need for the week. Organize the list by categories such as produce, dairy, protein, and pantry staples to make shopping more efficient.

5. Stick to the Perimeter:

- When grocery shopping, focus on the perimeter of the store where fresh produce, meats, dairy, and whole foods are typically located. Limit your time in the aisles where processed and packaged foods are found.

Batch Cooking and Freezing Meals for Convenience

Batch cooking and freezing meals in advance can save time and make it easier to stick to your meal plan during busy weeks. Here's how to do it effectively:

1. Choose Batch-Friendly Recipes:

- Look for recipes that are easily scalable and freeze well, such as soups, stews, casseroles, and chili. These dishes can be prepared in large batches and portioned out for future meals.

2. Schedule a Batch Cooking Session:

- Dedicate a few hours on a weekend or a day off to batch cook several meals at once. Cook multiple dishes simultaneously to maximize efficiency.

3. Invest in Storage Containers:

- Stock up on a variety of freezer-safe containers in different sizes to accommodate different portion sizes and meal types. Label containers with the contents and date of preparation for easy identification.

4. Portion Out Meals:

- Divide batch-cooked meals into individual portions before freezing to make it easier to grab and reheat single servings as needed. This helps prevent waste and allows for better portion control.

5. Rotate Your Freezer Stock:

- Keep track of what's in your freezer and rotate older meals to the front for quicker use. Use a "first in, first out" approach to ensure nothing goes to waste.

Strategies for Portion Control and Balanced Eating

Maintaining portion control is key to balanced eating and managing calorie intake. Here are some strategies to help you practice portion control effectively:

1. Use Smaller Plates and Bowls:

- Opt for smaller dinnerware to naturally reduce portion sizes. Research shows that people tend to eat less when they're served on smaller plates and bowls.

2. Fill Half Your Plate with Vegetables:

- Aim to fill at least half of your plate with non-starchy vegetables like leafy greens, broccoli, peppers, and carrots. This adds bulk and fiber to your meal without excess calories.

3. Measure Portions:

- Use measuring cups, spoons, and kitchen scales to portion out foods like grains, proteins, and fats. This helps you accurately control serving sizes and prevent overeating.

4. Practice Mindful Eating:

- Slow down and pay attention to your body's hunger and fullness cues while eating. Pause between bites, chew food thoroughly, and savor the flavors to prevent mindless overeating.

5. Be Mindful of Liquid Calories:

- Limit sugary beverages like soda, juice, and sweetened coffee drinks, which can contribute excess calories without providing satiety. Opt for water, unsweetened tea, or sparkling water with a splash of citrus instead.

Conclusion

Meal planning and preparation are essential tools for achieving success with your dietary goals. By implementing practical strategies for meal planning and grocery shopping, batch cooking and freezing meals, and practicing portion control and balanced eating, you can make healthier choices, save time, and stay on track with your nutrition plan. With consistency and dedication, meal planning and preparation can become habits that support your overall health and well-being for the long term.

CHPTER 12
31 DAYS MEAL PLAN

Week 1:

Day 1:

- Breakfast: Scrambled eggs with spinach and whole grain toast

- Snack: Greek yogurt with berries

- Lunch: Grilled chicken salad with mixed greens, cherry tomatoes, and balsamic vinaigrette

- Snack: Carrot sticks with hummus

- Dinner: Baked salmon with quinoa and roasted asparagus

Day 2:

- Breakfast: Oatmeal with sliced bananas and almonds

- Snack: Apple slices with peanut butter

- Lunch: Turkey and avocado wrap with lettuce and tomato

- Snack: Cottage cheese with pineapple chunks

- Dinner: Beef stir-fry with broccoli and brown rice

Day 3:

- Breakfast: Whole grain toast with almond butter and sliced strawberries

- Snack: Mixed nuts

- Lunch: Quinoa salad with black beans, corn, and bell peppers

- Snack: Celery sticks with cream cheese

- Dinner: Baked chicken breast with steamed green beans

Day 4:

- Breakfast: Greek yogurt with honey and walnuts

- Snack: Cottage cheese with cucumber slices

- Lunch: Tuna salad with mixed greens and lemon vinaigrette

- Snack: Cherry tomatoes with mozzarella cheese

- Dinner: Grilled shrimp skewers with zucchini noodles and marinara sauce

Day 5:

- Breakfast: Spinach and cheese omelette with whole grain toast

- Snack: Hard-boiled egg

- Lunch: Veggie wrap with hummus and sliced bell peppers

- Snack: Sliced bell peppers with guacamole

- Dinner: Baked cod with roasted Brussels sprouts

Day 6:

- Breakfast: Smoothie made with spinach, banana, and unsweetened almond milk

- Snack: Cottage cheese with pear slices

- Lunch: Turkey and cheese roll-ups with cucumber slices

- Snack: Almonds

- Dinner: Stir-fried tofu with mixed vegetables and quinoa

Day 7:

- Breakfast: Scrambled eggs with diced tomatoes and mushrooms

- Snack: Greek yogurt with berries

- Lunch: Grilled chicken Caesar salad with a light dressing

- Snack: Carrot sticks with hummus

- Dinner: Beef and broccoli stir-fry with brown rice

Week 2:

Day 8:

- Breakfast: Oatmeal with sliced apples and cinnamon

- Snack: Mixed nuts

- Lunch: Turkey and avocado wrap with lettuce and tomato

- Snack: Cottage cheese with pineapple chunks

- Dinner: Baked salmon with quinoa and roasted asparagus

Day 9:

- Breakfast: Whole grain toast with almond butter and banana slices

- Snack: Apple slices with peanut butter

- Lunch: Quinoa salad with black beans, corn, and bell peppers

- Snack: Celery sticks with cream cheese

- Dinner: Grilled chicken breast with steamed broccoli

Day 10:

- Breakfast: Greek yogurt with honey and walnuts

- Snack: Cottage cheese with cucumber slices

- Lunch: Tuna salad with mixed greens and lemon vinaigrette

- Snack: Cherry tomatoes with mozzarella cheese

- Dinner: Beef stir-fry with broccoli and brown rice

Day 11:

- Breakfast: Spinach and cheese omelette with whole grain toast

- Snack: Hard-boiled egg

- Lunch: Veggie wrap with hummus and sliced bell peppers

- Snack: Sliced bell peppers with guacamole

- Dinner: Baked cod with roasted Brussels sprouts

Day 12:

- Breakfast: Smoothie made with spinach, banana, and unsweetened almond milk

- Snack: Cottage cheese with pear slices

- Lunch: Turkey and cheese roll-ups with cucumber slices

- Snack: Almonds

- Dinner: Grilled shrimp skewers with zucchini noodles and marinara sauce

Day 13:

- Breakfast: Scrambled eggs with diced tomatoes and mushrooms

- Snack: Greek yogurt with berries

- Lunch: Grilled chicken Caesar salad with a light dressing

- Snack: Carrot sticks with hummus

- Dinner: Stir-fried tofu with mixed vegetables and quinoa

Day 14:

- Breakfast: Oatmeal with sliced apples and cinnamon

- Snack: Mixed nuts

- Lunch: Turkey and avocado wrap with lettuce and tomato

- Snack: Cottage cheese with pineapple chunks

- Dinner: Baked salmon with quinoa and roasted asparagus

Week 3:

Day 15:

- Breakfast: Whole grain toast with almond butter and banana slices

- Snack: Apple slices with peanut butter

- Lunch: Quinoa salad with black beans, corn, and bell peppers

- Snack: Celery sticks with cream cheese

- Dinner: Baked chicken breast with steamed green beans

Day 16:

- Breakfast: Greek yogurt with honey and walnuts

- Snack: Cottage cheese with cucumber slices

- Lunch: Tuna salad with mixed greens and lemon vinaigrette

- Snack: Cherry tomatoes with mozzarella cheese

- Dinner: Beef and broccoli stir-fry with brown rice

Day 17:

- Breakfast: Spinach and cheese omelette with whole grain toast

- Snack: Hard-boiled egg

- Lunch: Veggie wrap with hummus and sliced bell peppers

- Snack: Sliced bell peppers with guacamole

- Dinner: Baked cod with roasted Brussels sprouts

Day 18:

- Breakfast: Smoothie made with spinach, banana, and unsweetened almond milk

- Snack: Cottage cheese with pear slices

- Lunch: Turkey and cheese roll-ups with cucumber slices

- Snack: Almonds

- Dinner: Grilled shrimp skewers with zucchini noodles and marinara sauce

Day 19:

- Breakfast: Scrambled eggs with diced tomatoes and mushrooms

- Snack: Greek yogurt with berries

- Lunch: Grilled chicken Caesar salad with a light dressing

- Snack: Carrot sticks with hummus

- Dinner: Stir-fried tofu with mixed vegetables and quinoa

Day 20:

- Breakfast: Oatmeal with sliced apples and cinnamon

- Snack: Mixed nuts

- Lunch: Turkey and avocado wrap with lettuce and tomato

- Snack: Cottage cheese with pineapple chunks

- Dinner: Baked salmon with quinoa and roasted asparagus

Day 21:

- Breakfast: Whole grain toast with almond butter and banana slices

- Snack: Apple slices with peanut butter

- Lunch: Quinoa salad with black beans, corn, and bell peppers

- Snack: Celery sticks with cream cheese

- Dinner: Grilled chicken breast with steamed broccoli

Week 4:

Day 22:

- Breakfast: Greek yogurt with honey and walnuts

- Snack: Cottage cheese with cucumber slices

- Lunch: Tuna salad with mixed greens and lemon vinaigrette

- Snack: Cherry tomatoes with mozzarella cheese

- Dinner: Beef stir-fry with broccoli and brown rice

Day 23:

- Breakfast: Spinach and cheese omelette with whole grain toast

- Snack: Hard-boiled egg

- Lunch: Veggie wrap with hummus and sliced bell peppers

- Snack: Sliced bell peppers with guacamole

- Dinner: Baked cod with roasted Brussels sprouts

Day 24:

- Breakfast: Smoothie made with spinach, banana, and unsweetened almond milk

- Snack: Cottage cheese with pear slices

- Lunch: Turkey and cheese roll-ups with cucumber slices

- Snack: Almonds

- Dinner: Grilled shrimp skewers with zucchini noodles and marinara sauce

Day 25:

- Breakfast: Scrambled eggs with diced tomatoes and mushrooms

- Snack: Greek yogurt with berries

- Lunch: Grilled chicken Caesar salad with a light dressing

- Snack: Carrot sticks with hummus

- Dinner: Stir-fried tofu with mixed vegetables and quinoa

Day 26:

- Breakfast: Oatmeal with sliced apples and cinnamon

- Snack: Mixed nuts

- Lunch: Turkey and avocado wrap with lettuce and tomato

- Snack: Cottage cheese with pineapple chunks

- Dinner: Baked salmon with quinoa and roasted asparagus

Day 27:

- Breakfast: Whole grain toast with almond butter and banana slices
- Snack: Apple slices with peanut butter
- Lunch: Quinoa salad with black beans, corn, and bell peppers
- Snack: Celery sticks with cream cheese
- Dinner: Baked chicken breast with steamed green beans

Day 28:

- Breakfast: Greek yogurt with honey and walnuts
- Snack: Cottage cheese with cucumber slices
- Lunch: Tuna salad with mixed greens and lemon vinaigrette
- Snack: Cherry tomatoes with mozzarella cheese
- Dinner: Beef and broccoli stir-fry with brown rice

Day 29:

- Breakfast: Spinach and cheese omelette with whole grain toast
- Snack: Hard-boiled egg
- Lunch: Veggie wrap with hummus and sliced bell peppers

- Snack: Sliced bell peppers with guacamole

- Dinner: Baked cod with roasted Brussels sprouts

Day 30:

- Breakfast: Smoothie made with spinach, banana, and unsweetened almond milk

- Snack: Cottage cheese with pear slices

- Lunch: Turkey and cheese roll-ups with cucumber slices

- Snack: Almonds

- Dinner: Grilled shrimp skewers with zucchini noodles and marinara sauce

Day 31:

- Breakfast: Scrambled eggs with diced tomatoes and mushrooms

- Snack: Greek yogurt with berries

- Lunch: Grilled chicken Caesar salad with a light dressing

- Snack: Carrot sticks with hummus

- Dinner: Stir-fried tofu with mixed vegetables and quinoa

THE END